Good life

PCOS JOURNAL & TRACKER

"Everyday is a struggle but don't stop until you're proud"

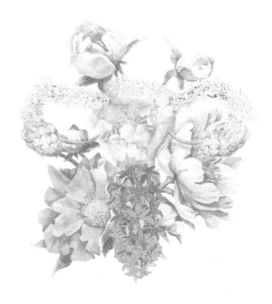

Dear Cyster,

Congratulations on taking a step towards healing your PCOS. **Good life PCOS Journal & tracker** is beautifully designed to support both your physical and mental health. It's a valuable tool in your PCOS journey to track your PCOS progress, Find out patterns & come up with your personalised diet and workout plan. The concept of "one size fits all" does not apply to healing PCOS. Everyone needs a holistic and personalized treatment plan. A journal or tracker can help you figure that out. Healing PCOS requires you to make healthy lifestyle changes. Consistency and commitment is a key to achieve that and this journal can help to incorporate healthy daily habits into your life. 5 major life style changes that need to be made for healing PCOS is healthy diet, exercise, stress management, proper sleep and remove environmental toxins. Apart from exercise and diet you can track your mood, sleep patterns, periods, weight log, water intake, energy levels, keep tab of supplements and medication & record your symptoms/side effects/cravings. This journal or tracker can be a life changer on your PCOS journey.

In my PCOS journey, tracking these changes and correlating with the symptoms really helped me in my healing process. It helped me figure out what supplements, workout, diet and stress management methods to follow. Having this in mind I designed this bullet journal. I am a independent researcher, a PCOS warrior, a youtuber and a influencer. I am helping and motivating cysters fight PCOS naturally through healthy lifestyle using social media. Feel free to join me there to know more about healing PCOS naturally.

Hope you use this journal well and reap the health benefits.

Good luck

Dr. D. Sherlin PhD.,
PCOS Cyster
Instagram : @good_life_hub
Youtube : goodlifehub

HOW THIS JOURNAL & TRACKER CAN HELP YOU IN YOUR PCOS HEALING JOURNEY

In addition to the brief letter on how this journal can help you. Here are few other ways this journal can aide you

- *It gives you the power to take control of your health.*
- *Increases self awareness: Writing down what you're doing and eating, holds you accountable to yourself. You become more aware.*
- *It will help to make healthy eating and wellness part of your regular routine*
- *It helps to find whether the changes you are making to your diet and lifestyle are improving your symptoms or not.*
- *It helps to figure out your own personalised diet plan and workout plan.*
- *It helps to track your PCOS progress and your journey. It gives motivation to know how far you have come and how much your symptoms have reduced. It's a motivational tool*
- *Helps you to listen to your body and make changes accordingly.*

IMPORTANCE OF EACH OF THE ENTRIES IN THE BULLET JOURNAL

1. ***Menstrual cycle and flow:*** *Your PCOS health directly reflects on your periods. The more your periods are becoming regular you know that your going on the right track and your healing your PCOS*
2. ***Mood*** *: It is a measure of your mental health. It can help you find out whether the stress management methods and other lifestyle changes are making a impact on your mental heath or not.*
3. ***Sleep*** *is very important for healing PCOS. Not just the quantity but also the quality of sleep. The goals should be to get 7-8 hrs sleep. You can also see the changes in your symptoms when you try to get a proper sleep*
4. ***Gratitude and mindfulness/meditation*** *is a great tool for stress management and helps to increase happiness and positive mindset.*

5. **Food log :** *Diet is the important medicine when it comes to healing PCOS. Having a food log can help in number of ways, helps to find food sensitivities (gluten, diary), when you are making a diet change you want to know how it affects your symptoms and your mental health. Does your diet helps to reduce weight ? Or increases weight? Whether your diet plan works or not?. This space can also be used for meal planning*

6. **Nutrition check list :** *For a healthy diet, it is recommended to have 4 proteins, 3 veggies, 2 fruits, 2 carbs, 4 tbsp nuts and 2tbsp seeds a day. Try to have a meal plan close to this nutrition. Seeds and nuts are very beneficial to healing PCOS so don't skip on that.*

7. **Water intake :** *Your water intake affects your energy, metabolism, weight loss, flushes toxins, removes craving and more. It is important to have at least 2L of water that is 8 glasses.*

8. **Weight log:** *helps to find if your workout and diet plan is helping you to reduce weight. If reducing weight is not your goal or you get depressed seeing your weight everyday. just skip this!*

9. **Workout plan** *: Exercise or any physical exercise is a must in the healing process. Do any physical activity that you like! Change your physical activity as per your liking and energy! Writing down your exercise plan can help you figure out which workout routine works best for you*

10. **Supplements and medicine** *: There are lot of supplement for PCOS. Not everything is helpful some really doesn't do anything at all. It is advisable to try one supplements at a time so that you know how it affects your symptoms. Take a supplement for at least 2 months to see the benefits. If your taking any medicines you need to know whether it is causing any side effects or not , having a log helps with that*

11. **Energy level** *: Lot of women with PCOS suffer from chronic fatigue. This is an indicator of how your workout and diet is fuelling your body.*

12. **Symptoms and response**: *This is a very important field. Write down every symptom you experience. Mentally and physically. Every action you take for healing PCOS needs to be correlated with this to know your PCOS progress and for making any change.*

HOW TO USE THIS PCOS BULLET JOURNAL

To effectively use the journal, Fill out date, sleep log, gratitude and weight in the morning. Fill rest of the journal at night

1. *Write down the date* **DATE:** 7/8/20

2. *Write your cycle day, next to it there is tear shaped box. Colour it if you have your periods on that day. You can also indicate the amount of flow in the box- fully colouring it to indicate heavy flow, colour till half to indicate normal or colouring it near the bottom to indicate scanty flow. Use the way you want, you can also use different colours to fill.*

    CYCLE DAY : 3 🌢

3. *Tick out the mood for the day. How you felt on an average. From very happy, happy, neutral, sad and depressed.*

    MOOD: 😊😊😐😟😣

4. *Write down the sleep hours and the total hours you have slept. Your goal should be to reach an average of 7-8 hrs sleep.*

    🌙💤 **SLEPT FROM** 10:00 **TO** 6:15   **TOTAL HOURS:** 8hr 15 min.

5. *Write three things you are grateful for; writing gratitude helps to improve your mood and kick-start your day with a positive mindset. You can even write more than three things to be thankful for.*

    I AM THANKFUL FOR ... 🙏
    1. a productive day, uploaded video
    2. completed decluttering kitchen
    3. beautiful weather

6. *Indicate your water intake by shading the number of glasses you drank during the day. Your goal should be min. of 8 glasses.*

    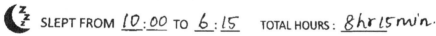
    Water: 🥛🥛🥛🥛🥛🥛⬜⬜⬜⬜⬜

7. *Write your Food log; you can also use this for meal planning. Write everything that you eat. There is also a Nutrition check list so keep that in mind while planning your meals.*

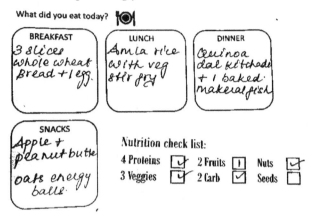

What did you eat today?

BREAKFAST
3 slices whole wheat Bread + 1 egg.

LUNCH
Amla rice with veg stir fry

DINNER
Quinoa dal kitchadi + 1 baked makeral fish

SNACKS
Apple + peanut butter
oats energy balls.

Nutrition check list:
4 Proteins	☑	2 Fruits	☑	Nuts	☑
3 Veggies	☑	2 Carb	☑	Seeds	☐

8. *If you meditated or followed any mindfulness exercise, Tick the mindfulness check box.*
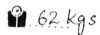 : ☑

9. *Record your weight. Its best to record weight at the same time everyday.*

62 kgs

10. *Record your workout routine. You can also use this space to plan your workout for the day. It can be yoga, simple exercises or any physical activity. Write the number of reps and sets you did.*

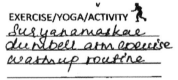

EXERCISE/YOGA/ACTIVITY
Suryanamaskar
dumbell arm exercise
warmup routine

11. *Supplements and medicine log. Write the medicines and the supplements you took during the day. Write the dosage and also the number of capsules/tab you took*

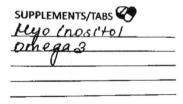

SUPPLEMENTS/TABS
Myo Inositol
omega 3

12. *Fill in your energy levels. There are three blocks in the battery shaped box. If you had low energy shade only the first box, If your energy was okay colour first two and if you had high energy shade all the three blocks.*

13. *The last and the very important field to record is the symptoms, cravings and the side affects you experienced during the day. Write as per your needs but to help with filling this field I have given a list of symptoms commonly experienced by PCOS women in the next page. You can make a bookmark with it and use it as a guide to fill the symptoms.*

SYMPTOMS/CRAVINGS/RESPONSE

Headache, mood swing, pain legs, fatigue.

It is advisable to use this journal for a minimum of 6-8 months to see visible results in your health. Depending on the individual needs it takes time to figure out your own diet, workout, stress management methods and supplements. There is no "quick fix" for PCOS, healing PCOS is a process and this journal is a valuable tool in helping you overcome PCOS.

I have given a blank page in the beginning to write down your goals. what you wish to achieve in this 3 month. What is your plan of action. What supplements, workout plan and diet you going to implement. You can also use this space for writing affirmations to help you achieve your PCOS goals. At the end of the journal, I have given 3 blank pages to help you assess the progress you have made. Go through the journal and see which changes are helping you in a positive way.

Use the journal in the best possible way for your health. Don't forget to leave a review in the amazon product page. How you felt after seeing this journal ? About the entries, description and the cover look. How it was helpful? Do you wish for any changes in the upcoming version?

Good luck with the journal !

A Bookmark to guide you with writing your symptoms & motivate you

If you bite it
Write it
If you drink it
Ink it
If you feel it
Scribble it

Strive for Progress not Perfection

Insomnia
Confusion
Brain fog
Headache
Dizziness
Breast pain
Body aches
Gas
Hot flashes
Chills
PMS
Spotting
Nausea
Vomiting
Diarrhoea
Constipation
Abdominal pain
Acidity
Acid reflux
Stress
Moodiness
Irritability
Tension
Hair fall level
Hirsutism level

Write down your Goals / affirmations
/ Motivational quotes

DATE: _____ CYCLE DAY : ☐ ⬭ MOOD: 😄 🙂 😐 🙁 😣

🌙 SLEPT FROM ___:___ TO ___:___   TOTAL HOURS : _____

I AM THANKFUL FOR ... 🙏

1._____
2._____
3._____

What did you eat today? 🍽️

BREAKFAST	LUNCH	DINNER

SNACKS

Nutrition check list:

4 Proteins ☐   2 Fruits ☐   Nuts ☐
3 Veggies ☐   2 Carb ☐   Seeds ☐

Water: ▯▯▯▯▯▯▯▯▯▯

🧘 : ☐   ⚖️

SUPPLEMENTS/TABS 💊   EXERCISE/YOGA/ACTIVITY 🏃

_____   _____
_____   _____
_____   _____
_____   _____
_____   _____

SYMPTOMS/CRAVINGS/RESPONSE 🧍   ⚡ 🔋▮▮▮

_____
_____
_____

DATE: _____ CYCLE DAY : ☐ ◇ MOOD: 😃 ☺ 😐 ☹ 😣

🌙 SLEPT FROM ___:___ TO ___:___ TOTAL HOURS : _____

I AM THANKFUL FOR ... 🙏

1._____
2._____
3._____

What did you eat today? 🍽

BREAKFAST	LUNCH	DINNER

SNACKS	Nutrition check list:
	4 Proteins ☐ 2 Fruits ☐ Nuts ☐
	3 Veggies ☐ 2 Carb ☐ Seeds ☐

Water: ⬜⬜⬜⬜⬜⬜⬜⬜⬜⬜

🧘 : ☐   ⚖ ....

SUPPLEMENTS/TABS 💊   EXERCISE/YOGA/ACTIVITY 🏃

_____   _____
_____   _____
_____   _____
_____   _____
_____   _____

SYMPTOMS/CRAVINGS/RESPONSE 🧍   ⚡ 🔋

_____
_____
_____

DATE: _____ CYCLE DAY : ☐ ⬭ MOOD: 😀 🙂 😐 🙁 😣

🌙💤 SLEPT FROM ___:___ TO ___:___ TOTAL HOURS : _____

I AM THANKFUL FOR ... 🙏
1._____
2._____
3._____

What did you eat today? 🍽

BREAKFAST	LUNCH	DINNER

SNACKS

Nutrition check list:

4 Proteins ☐   2 Fruits ☐   Nuts ☐
3 Veggies ☐   2 Carb ☐   Seeds ☐

Water: 🥛🥛🥛🥛🥛🥛🥛🥛🥛🥛🥛

🧘 : ☐   ⚖ _____

SUPPLEMENTS/TABS 💊   EXERCISE/YOGA/ACTIVITY 🏃

_____   _____
_____   _____
_____   _____
_____   _____
_____   _____

SYMPTOMS/CRAVINGS/RESPONSE 🧍   ⚡ 🔋

_____
_____
_____

DATE: _____ CYCLE DAY : [   ] 🌢 MOOD: 😀 🙂 😐 🙁 😫

🌙 SLEPT FROM ___:___ TO ___:___ TOTAL HOURS : _____

I AM THANKFUL FOR ... 🙏

1._____
2._____
3._____

What did you eat today? 🍽

BREAKFAST	LUNCH	DINNER

SNACKS	Nutrition check list:

Nutrition check list:

4 Proteins [ ] 2 Fruits [ ] Nuts [ ]
3 Veggies [ ] 2 Carb [ ] Seeds [ ]

Water: 🥛🥛🥛🥛🥛🥛🥛🥛🥛🥛🥛

🧘 : [ ]   ⚖ ....

SUPPLEMENTS/TABS 💊

_____
_____
_____
_____

EXERCISE/YOGA/ACTIVITY 🏃

_____
_____
_____
_____

SYMPTOMS/CRAVINGS/RESPONSE 🧍   ⚡ [■■]

_____
_____
_____

DATE: _____ CYCLE DAY : [ ] ⬡ MOOD: 😃 🙂 😐 🙁 😫

🌙 SLEPT FROM ___:___ TO ___:___ TOTAL HOURS : _____

I AM THANKFUL FOR ... 🙏

1. _____
2. _____
3. _____

What did you eat today? 🍽

BREAKFAST	LUNCH	DINNER

SNACKS

Nutrition check list:

| 4 Proteins [ ] | 2 Fruits [ ] | Nuts [ ] |
| 3 Veggies [ ] | 2 Carb [ ] | Seeds [ ] |

Water: 🥛🥛🥛🥛🥛🥛🥛🥛🥛🥛

🧘 : [ ]   ⚖️

SUPPLEMENTS/TABS 💊   EXERCISE/YOGA/ACTIVITY 🏃

_____   _____
_____   _____
_____   _____
_____   _____
_____   _____

SYMPTOMS/CRAVINGS/RESPONSE 🧍   ⚡ 🔋

_____
_____
_____

DATE: _____ CYCLE DAY : ☐ ⬦ MOOD: 😀 🙂 😐 🙁 😣

🌙💤 SLEPT FROM ___:___ TO ___:___ TOTAL HOURS : _____

I AM THANKFUL FOR ... 🙏
1. _____
2. _____
3. _____

What did you eat today? 🍽️

BREAKFAST	LUNCH	DINNER

SNACKS	Nutrition check list:

Nutrition check list:

4 Proteins ☐   2 Fruits ☐   Nuts ☐
3 Veggies ☐   2 Carb ☐   Seeds ☐

Water: 🥛🥛🥛🥛🥛🥛🥛🥛🥛🥛🥛

🧘 : ☐   ⚖️

SUPPLEMENTS/TABS 💊   EXERCISE/YOGA/ACTIVITY 🏃
_____   _____
_____   _____
_____   _____
_____   _____
_____   _____

SYMPTOMS/CRAVINGS/RESPONSE 🧍   ⚡ 🔋
_____
_____
_____

DATE: _____   CYCLE DAY : [　] ⬭   MOOD: 😃 🙂 😐 🙁 😣

🌙 SLEPT FROM ___:___ TO ___:___   TOTAL HOURS : _____

I AM THANKFUL FOR ... 🙏
1._____
2._____
3._____

What did you eat today? 🍽

BREAKFAST	LUNCH	DINNER

SNACKS	Nutrition check list:

Nutrition check list:

4 Proteins [　]   2 Fruits [　]   Nuts [　]
3 Veggies [　]   2 Carb [　]   Seeds [　]

Water: 🥤🥤🥤🥤🥤🥤🥤🥤🥤🥤

🧘 : [　]   ⚖ _____

SUPPLEMENTS/TABS 💊   EXERCISE/YOGA/ACTIVITY 🏃

_____   _____
_____   _____
_____   _____
_____   _____
_____   _____

SYMPTOMS/CRAVINGS/RESPONSE 🔍   ⚡ [　][　][　]

_____
_____
_____

DATE: _____ CYCLE DAY : ☐ ◊ MOOD: 😀 😊 😐 🙁 ☹️

SLEPT FROM ___:___ TO ___:___ TOTAL HOURS : _____

I AM THANKFUL FOR ...

1._____
2._____
3._____

What did you eat today?

BREAKFAST	LUNCH	DINNER

SNACKS

Nutrition check list:

4 Proteins ☐   2 Fruits ☐   Nuts ☐
3 Veggies ☐   2 Carb ☐   Seeds ☐

Water: ⊔⊔⊔⊔⊔⊔⊔⊔⊔⊔⊔⊔

🧘 : ☐

SUPPLEMENTS/TABS

_____
_____
_____
_____
_____

EXERCISE/YOGA/ACTIVITY

_____
_____
_____
_____
_____

SYMPTOMS/CRAVINGS/RESPONSE ⚡ 🔋

_____
_____
_____

DATE: _____ CYCLE DAY : [ ] ⬡ MOOD: 😊 🙂 😐 🙁 😣

🌙 SLEPT FROM ___:___ TO ___:___ TOTAL HOURS : _____

I AM THANKFUL FOR ... 🙏
1._____
2._____
3._____

What did you eat today? 🍽️

BREAKFAST	LUNCH	DINNER

SNACKS	Nutrition check list:

Nutrition check list:

4 Proteins [ ]   2 Fruits [ ]   Nuts [ ]
3 Veggies [ ]   2 Carb [ ]   Seeds [ ]

Water: 🥛🥛🥛🥛🥛🥛🥛🥛🥛🥛🥛

🧘 : [ ]   ⚖️ _____

SUPPLEMENTS/TABS 💊
_____
_____
_____
_____
_____

EXERCISE/YOGA/ACTIVITY 🏃
_____
_____
_____
_____
_____

SYMPTOMS/CRAVINGS/RESPONSE 🧍   ⚡ 🔋
_____
_____
_____

DATE: _____ CYCLE DAY : ☐ ⬥ MOOD: 😊 🙂 😐 🙁 😫

🌙💤 SLEPT FROM ___:___ TO ___:___ TOTAL HOURS : _____

I AM THANKFUL FOR ... 🙏
1._____
2._____
3._____

What did you eat today? 🍽️

BREAKFAST	LUNCH	DINNER

SNACKS

Nutrition check list:

4 Proteins ☐ 2 Fruits ☐ Nuts ☐
3 Veggies ☐ 2 Carb ☐ Seeds ☐

Water: 🥛🥛🥛🥛🥛🥛🥛🥛🥛🥛🥛

🧘 : ☐   ⚖️

SUPPLEMENTS/TABS 💊

_____
_____
_____
_____

EXERCISE/YOGA/ACTIVITY 🏃

_____
_____
_____
_____

SYMPTOMS/CRAVINGS/RESPONSE 🧍   ⚡ 🔋

_____
_____
_____

DATE: _____ CYCLE DAY : ☐ ◊ MOOD: 😃 🙂 😐 🙁 😫

🌙💤 SLEPT FROM ___:___ TO ___:___ TOTAL HOURS : _____

I AM THANKFUL FOR ... 🙏

1._____
2._____
3._____

What did you eat today? 🍽

BREAKFAST	LUNCH	DINNER

SNACKS

Nutrition check list:

4 Proteins ☐   2 Fruits ☐   Nuts ☐
3 Veggies ☐   2 Carb ☐   Seeds ☐

Water: ☐☐☐☐☐☐☐☐☐☐☐

🧘 : ☐   👝

SUPPLEMENTS/TABS 💊

_____
_____
_____
_____
_____

EXERCISE/YOGA/ACTIVITY 🏃

_____
_____
_____
_____
_____

SYMPTOMS/CRAVINGS/RESPONSE 🧍   ⚡ 🔋

_____
_____
_____

DATE: _____ CYCLE DAY : ☐ 💧 MOOD: 😄 🙂 😐 🙁 😣

🌙💤 SLEPT FROM ___:___ TO ___:___ TOTAL HOURS : _____

I AM THANKFUL FOR ... 🙏
1. _____
2. _____
3. _____

What did you eat today? 🍽

BREAKFAST	LUNCH	DINNER

SNACKS

Nutrition check list:

| 4 Proteins ☐ | 2 Fruits ☐ | Nuts ☐ |
| 3 Veggies ☐ | 2 Carb ☐ | Seeds ☐ |

Water: 🥛🥛🥛🥛🥛🥛🥛🥛🥛🥛🥛

🧘 : ☐   ⚖

SUPPLEMENTS/TABS 💊

EXERCISE/YOGA/ACTIVITY 🏃

_____   _____
_____   _____
_____   _____
_____   _____
_____   _____

SYMPTOMS/CRAVINGS/RESPONSE 🧍   ⚡ 🔋

_____
_____
_____

DATE: _____ CYCLE DAY : ☐ ⬭ MOOD: 😀 🙂 😐 🙁 😫

🌙 SLEPT FROM ___:___ TO ___:___ TOTAL HOURS : _____

I AM THANKFUL FOR ... 🙏

1._____
2._____
3._____

What did you eat today? 🍽️

BREAKFAST	LUNCH	DINNER

SNACKS

Nutrition check list:

4 Proteins ☐   2 Fruits ☐   Nuts ☐
3 Veggies ☐   2 Carb ☐   Seeds ☐

Water: 🥛🥛🥛🥛🥛🥛🥛🥛🥛🥛

🧘 : ☐   ⚖️ ....

SUPPLEMENTS/TABS 💊   EXERCISE/YOGA/ACTIVITY 🏃

_____   _____
_____   _____
_____   _____
_____   _____
_____   _____

SYMPTOMS/CRAVINGS/RESPONSE 🔍   ⚡ 🔋

_____
_____
_____

DATE: _____   CYCLE DAY : [____] ⬦   MOOD: 😀 🙂 😐 🙁 😣

🌙💤 SLEPT FROM ___:___ TO ___:___   TOTAL HOURS : _____

I AM THANKFUL FOR ... 🙏

1._____
2._____
3._____

What did you eat today? 🍽️

BREAKFAST	LUNCH	DINNER

SNACKS

Nutrition check list:

| 4 Proteins ☐ | 2 Fruits ☐ | Nuts ☐ |
| 3 Veggies ☐ | 2 Carb ☐ | Seeds ☐ |

Water: 🥛🥛🥛🥛🥛🥛🥛🥛🥛🥛🥛🥛

🧘 : ☐   ⚖️ _____

SUPPLEMENTS/TABS 💊

EXERCISE/YOGA/ACTIVITY 🏃

_____   _____
_____   _____
_____   _____
_____   _____
_____   _____

SYMPTOMS/CRAVINGS/RESPONSE 🧍   ⚡ 🔋

_____
_____
_____

DATE: _____ CYCLE DAY : [ ] 🜄 MOOD: 😐 🙂 😕 🙁 😣

🌙 SLEPT FROM ___:___ TO ___:___ TOTAL HOURS : _____

I AM THANKFUL FOR ... 🙏

1. _____
2. _____
3. _____

What did you eat today? 🍽️

BREAKFAST	LUNCH	DINNER

SNACKS

Nutrition check list:

4 Proteins [ ]	2 Fruits [ ]	Nuts [ ]
3 Veggies [ ]	2 Carb [ ]	Seeds [ ]

Water: 🥛🥛🥛🥛🥛🥛🥛🥛🥛🥛🥛

🧘 : [ ]   ⚖️ ....

SUPPLEMENTS/TABS 💊

_____
_____
_____
_____
_____

EXERCISE/YOGA/ACTIVITY 🏃

_____
_____
_____
_____
_____

SYMPTOMS/CRAVINGS/RESPONSE 🧍   ⚡ 🔋

_____
_____
_____

DATE: _____   CYCLE DAY : [ ]   ⬭   MOOD: 😊 🙂 😐 🙁 😣

🌙💤 SLEPT FROM ___:___ TO ___:___   TOTAL HOURS : _____

I AM THANKFUL FOR ... 🙏
1. _____
2. _____
3. _____

What did you eat today? 🍽

BREAKFAST	LUNCH	DINNER

SNACKS	Nutrition check list:

Nutrition check list:

4 Proteins [ ]	2 Fruits [ ]	Nuts [ ]
3 Veggies [ ]	2 Carb [ ]	Seeds [ ]

Water: 🥛🥛🥛🥛🥛🥛🥛🥛🥛🥛

🧘 : [ ]   ⚖

SUPPLEMENTS/TABS 💊
_____
_____
_____
_____
_____

EXERCISE/YOGA/ACTIVITY 🏃
_____
_____
_____
_____
_____

SYMPTOMS/CRAVINGS/RESPONSE 🧍   ⚡ 🔋
_____
_____
_____

DATE: _____ CYCLE DAY : [ ] ⬦ MOOD: 😃 🙂 😐 🙁 😣

🌙 SLEPT FROM ___:___ TO ___:___ TOTAL HOURS : _____

I AM THANKFUL FOR ... 🙏

1. _____
2. _____
3. _____

What did you eat today? 🍽️

BREAKFAST	LUNCH	DINNER

SNACKS

Nutrition check list:

| 4 Proteins [ ] | 2 Fruits [ ] | Nuts [ ] |
| 3 Veggies [ ] | 2 Carb [ ] | Seeds [ ] |

Water: 🥛🥛🥛🥛🥛🥛🥛🥛🥛🥛🥛

🧘 : [ ]   ⚖️

SUPPLEMENTS/TABS 💊   EXERCISE/YOGA/ACTIVITY 🏃

_____   _____
_____   _____
_____   _____
_____   _____
_____   _____

SYMPTOMS/CRAVINGS/RESPONSE 🧍   ⚡ 🔋

_____
_____
_____

DATE: _____ CYCLE DAY : ☐ ◇ MOOD: 😀 🙂 😐 🙁 😣

🌙 💤 SLEPT FROM ___:___ TO ___:___ TOTAL HOURS : _____

I AM THANKFUL FOR ... 🙏
1. _____
2. _____
3. _____

What did you eat today? 🍽

BREAKFAST	LUNCH	DINNER

SNACKS	Nutrition check list:

Nutrition check list:

4 Proteins ☐   2 Fruits ☐   Nuts ☐
3 Veggies ☐   2 Carb ☐   Seeds ☐

Water: 🥛🥛🥛🥛🥛🥛🥛🥛🥛🥛🥛🥛

🧘 : ☐   ⚖ _____

SUPPLEMENTS/TABS 💊   EXERCISE/YOGA/ACTIVITY 🏃

_____   _____
_____   _____
_____   _____
_____   _____

SYMPTOMS/CRAVINGS/RESPONSE 🧍   ⚡ 🔋

_____
_____
_____

DATE: _____ CYCLE DAY : ☐ ⬡ MOOD: 😀 🙂 😐 ☹️ 😣

🌙 SLEPT FROM ___:___ TO ___:___ TOTAL HOURS : _____

I AM THANKFUL FOR ... 🙏
1._____
2._____
3._____

What did you eat today? 🍽️

BREAKFAST	LUNCH	DINNER

SNACKS

Nutrition check list:

4 Proteins ☐   2 Fruits ☐   Nuts ☐
3 Veggies ☐   2 Carb ☐   Seeds ☐

Water: ▭▭▭▭▭▭▭▭▭▭

🧘 : ☐   ⚖️

SUPPLEMENTS/TABS 💊

_____
_____
_____
_____
_____

EXERCISE/YOGA/ACTIVITY 🏃

_____
_____
_____
_____

SYMPTOMS/CRAVINGS/RESPONSE 🧍   ⚡ 🔋

_____
_____
_____

DATE: _____ CYCLE DAY : [ ] ⬦ MOOD: 🙂😊😐🙁😞

🌙 SLEPT FROM ___:___ TO ___:___ TOTAL HOURS : _____

I AM THANKFUL FOR ... 🙏
1._____
2._____
3._____

What did you eat today? 🍽️

BREAKFAST	LUNCH	DINNER

SNACKS

Nutrition check list:

4 Proteins [ ]   2 Fruits [ ]   Nuts [ ]
3 Veggies [ ]   2 Carb [ ]   Seeds [ ]

Water: 🥛🥛🥛🥛🥛🥛🥛🥛🥛🥛🥛

🧘 : [ ]   ⚖️ ....

SUPPLEMENTS/TABS 💊

EXERCISE/YOGA/ACTIVITY 🏃

_____   _____
_____   _____
_____   _____
_____   _____
_____   _____

SYMPTOMS/CRAVINGS/RESPONSE 🧍   ⚡ 🔋

_____
_____
_____

DATE: _____   CYCLE DAY : ☐ ◊   MOOD: 😃 🙂 😐 🙁 😣

🌙 SLEPT FROM ___:___ TO ___:___   TOTAL HOURS : _____

I AM THANKFUL FOR ... 🙏

1._____
2._____
3._____

What did you eat today? 🍽

BREAKFAST	LUNCH	DINNER

SNACKS	Nutrition check list:

Nutrition check list:

4 Proteins ☐   2 Fruits ☐   Nuts ☐
3 Veggies ☐   2 Carb ☐   Seeds ☐

Water: ☐☐☐☐☐☐☐☐☐☐☐

🧘 : ☐   ⚖

SUPPLEMENTS/TABS 💊

_____
_____
_____
_____
_____

EXERCISE/YOGA/ACTIVITY 🏃

_____
_____
_____
_____

SYMPTOMS/CRAVINGS/RESPONSE 🧍   ⚡ 🔋

_____
_____
_____

DATE: _____ CYCLE DAY : ☐ ⬭ MOOD: 😊 🙂 😐 🙁 😣

🌙 SLEPT FROM ___:___ TO ___:___ TOTAL HOURS : _____

I AM THANKFUL FOR ... 🙏
1._____
2._____
3._____

What did you eat today? 🍽️

BREAKFAST	LUNCH	DINNER

SNACKS

Nutrition check list:

4 Proteins ☐   2 Fruits ☐   Nuts ☐
3 Veggies ☐   2 Carb ☐   Seeds ☐

Water: 🥛🥛🥛🥛🥛🥛🥛🥛🥛🥛

🧘 : ☐   ⏱️ _____

SUPPLEMENTS/TABS 💊   EXERCISE/YOGA/ACTIVITY 🏃

_____   _____
_____   _____
_____   _____
_____   _____
_____   _____

SYMPTOMS/CRAVINGS/RESPONSE 🧍   ⚡ 🔋▢▢

_____
_____
_____

DATE: _____ CYCLE DAY : [ ] ⬯ MOOD: 😛 🙂 😐 🙁 😫

🌙💤 SLEPT FROM ___:___ TO ___:___   TOTAL HOURS : _____

I AM THANKFUL FOR ... 🙏

1._____
2._____
3._____

What did you eat today? 🍽

BREAKFAST	LUNCH	DINNER

SNACKS	Nutrition check list:

Nutrition check list:

4 Proteins [ ]   2 Fruits [ ]   Nuts [ ]
3 Veggies [ ]   2 Carb [ ]   Seeds [ ]

Water: 🥛🥛🥛🥛🥛🥛🥛🥛🥛🥛

🧘 : [ ]   ⚖

SUPPLEMENTS/TABS 💊

_____   _____
_____   _____
_____   _____
_____   _____
_____   _____

EXERCISE/YOGA/ACTIVITY 🏃

SYMPTOMS/CRAVINGS/RESPONSE 🧍   ⚡ 🔋

_____
_____
_____

DATE: _____ CYCLE DAY : [ ] ⬭ MOOD: 😀 🙂 😐 🙁 😣

🌙💤 SLEPT FROM ___:___ TO ___:___ TOTAL HOURS : _____

I AM THANKFUL FOR ... 🙏

1. _____
2. _____
3. _____

What did you eat today? 🍽️

BREAKFAST	LUNCH	DINNER

SNACKS

Nutrition check list:

4 Proteins [ ]   2 Fruits [ ]   Nuts [ ]
3 Veggies [ ]   2 Carb [ ]   Seeds [ ]

Water: 🥛🥛🥛🥛🥛🥛🥛🥛🥛🥛

🧘 : [ ]   ⚖️ ....

SUPPLEMENTS/TABS 💊   EXERCISE/YOGA/ACTIVITY 🏃

_____   _____
_____   _____
_____   _____
_____   _____
_____   _____

SYMPTOMS/CRAVINGS/RESPONSE 🧍   ⚡ 🔋

_____
_____
_____

DATE: _____ CYCLE DAY : [   ] 🌢 MOOD: 😃 🙂 😐 ☹️ 😣

🌙 SLEPT FROM ___:___ TO ___:___   TOTAL HOURS : _____

I AM THANKFUL FOR ... 🙏

1._____
2._____
3._____

What did you eat today? 🍽️

BREAKFAST	LUNCH	DINNER

SNACKS	Nutrition check list:

Nutrition check list:

4 Proteins [ ]   2 Fruits [ ]   Nuts [ ]
3 Veggies [ ]   2 Carb [ ]   Seeds [ ]

Water: 🥛🥛🥛🥛🥛🥛🥛🥛🥛🥛🥛

🧘 : [ ]   ⚖️ _____

SUPPLEMENTS/TABS 💊   EXERCISE/YOGA/ACTIVITY 🏃

_____   _____
_____   _____
_____   _____
_____   _____
_____   _____

SYMPTOMS/CRAVINGS/RESPONSE 🧍   ⚡ 🔋

_____
_____
_____

DATE: _____ CYCLE DAY : [ ] ⬡ MOOD: 😀 🙂 😐 🙁 😫

🌙 SLEPT FROM ___:___ TO ___:___ TOTAL HOURS : _____

I AM THANKFUL FOR ... 🙏
1._____
2._____
3._____

What did you eat today? 🍽

BREAKFAST	LUNCH	DINNER

SNACKS	Nutrition check list:

Nutrition check list:

4 Proteins [ ]   2 Fruits [ ]   Nuts [ ]
3 Veggies [ ]   2 Carb [ ]   Seeds [ ]

Water: 🥤🥤🥤🥤🥤🥤🥤🥤🥤🥤🥤

🧘 : [ ]   ⚖ _____

SUPPLEMENTS/TABS 💊
_____
_____
_____
_____
_____

EXERCISE/YOGA/ACTIVITY 🏃
_____
_____
_____
_____
_____

SYMPTOMS/CRAVINGS/RESPONSE 🧍   ⚡ 🔋
_____
_____
_____

DATE: _____ CYCLE DAY : [ ] ⬡ MOOD: 😀 🙂 😐 🙁 ☹️

🌙💤 SLEPT FROM ___:___ TO ___:___ TOTAL HOURS : _____

I AM THANKFUL FOR ... 🙏

1._____

2._____

3._____

What did you eat today? 🍽️

BREAKFAST	LUNCH	DINNER

SNACKS

Nutrition check list:

4 Proteins [ ]   2 Fruits [ ]   Nuts [ ]

3 Veggies [ ]   2 Carb [ ]   Seeds [ ]

Water: 🥤🥤🥤🥤🥤🥤🥤🥤🥤🥤🥤

🧘 : [ ]   ⚖️

SUPPLEMENTS/TABS 💊

_____

_____

_____

_____

_____

EXERCISE/YOGA/ACTIVITY 🏃

_____

_____

_____

_____

_____

SYMPTOMS/CRAVINGS/RESPONSE 🧍   ⚡ 🔋

_____

_____

_____

DATE: _____ CYCLE DAY : ☐ ⬡ MOOD: 😄 🙂 😐 🙁 😣

🌙 SLEPT FROM ___:___ TO ___:___ TOTAL HOURS : _____

I AM THANKFUL FOR ... 🙏

1. _____
2. _____
3. _____

What did you eat today? 🍽️

BREAKFAST	LUNCH	DINNER

SNACKS	Nutrition check list:

Nutrition check list:

4 Proteins ☐   2 Fruits ☐   Nuts ☐
3 Veggies ☐   2 Carb ☐   Seeds ☐

Water: 🥛🥛🥛🥛🥛🥛🥛🥛🥛🥛

🧘 : ☐   ⚖️ _____

SUPPLEMENTS/TABS 💊

_____
_____
_____
_____

EXERCISE/YOGA/ACTIVITY 🏃

_____
_____
_____
_____

SYMPTOMS/CRAVINGS/RESPONSE 🧍   ⚡ 🔋

_____
_____
_____

DATE: _____ CYCLE DAY : ☐ ◯ MOOD: 😀😊😐😟😣

🌙 SLEPT FROM ___:___ TO ___:___ TOTAL HOURS : _____

I AM THANKFUL FOR ... 🙏

1._____
2._____
3._____

What did you eat today? 🍽️

BREAKFAST	LUNCH	DINNER

SNACKS

Nutrition check list:

4 Proteins ☐   2 Fruits ☐   Nuts ☐
3 Veggies ☐   2 Carb ☐   Seeds ☐

Water: 🥛🥛🥛🥛🥛🥛🥛🥛🥛🥛

🧘 : ☐   ⚖️ ....

SUPPLEMENTS/TABS 💊

_____
_____
_____
_____
_____

EXERCISE/YOGA/ACTIVITY 🏃

_____
_____
_____
_____
_____

SYMPTOMS/CRAVINGS/RESPONSE 🧍   ⚡ 🔋

_____
_____
_____

DATE: _____ CYCLE DAY : ☐ 💧 MOOD: 😃 🙂 😐 🙁 😖

🌙 SLEPT FROM ___:___ TO ___:___ TOTAL HOURS : _____

I AM THANKFUL FOR ... 🙏
1._____
2._____
3._____

What did you eat today? 🍽

BREAKFAST	LUNCH	DINNER

SNACKS

Nutrition check list:

| 4 Proteins ☐ | 2 Fruits ☐ | Nuts ☐ |
| 3 Veggies ☐ | 2 Carb ☐ | Seeds ☐ |

Water: 🥤🥤🥤🥤🥤🥤🥤🥤🥤🥤

🧘 : ☐   ⚖

SUPPLEMENTS/TABS 💊   EXERCISE/YOGA/ACTIVITY 🏃

_____   _____
_____   _____
_____   _____
_____   _____

SYMPTOMS/CRAVINGS/RESPONSE 🧍   ⚡ 🔋

_____
_____
_____

DATE: _____ CYCLE DAY : [ ] ⬦ MOOD: 😀 🙂 😐 🙁 😣

🌙 SLEPT FROM ___:___ TO ___:___ TOTAL HOURS : _____

I AM THANKFUL FOR ... 🙏

1._____
2._____
3._____

What did you eat today? 🍽️

BREAKFAST	LUNCH	DINNER

SNACKS

Nutrition check list:

4 Proteins [ ]   2 Fruits [ ]   Nuts [ ]
3 Veggies [ ]   2 Carb [ ]   Seeds [ ]

Water: ⬜⬜⬜⬜⬜⬜⬜⬜⬜⬜

🧘 : [ ]   ⚖️

SUPPLEMENTS/TABS 💊   EXERCISE/YOGA/ACTIVITY 🏃

_____   _____
_____   _____
_____   _____
_____   _____

SYMPTOMS/CRAVINGS/RESPONSE 🧍   ⚡ [▮▮▮]

_____
_____
_____

DATE: _____ CYCLE DAY : [ ] ⬭ MOOD: 😀 🙂 😐 🙁 😣

🌙 SLEPT FROM ___:___ TO ___:___ TOTAL HOURS : _____

I AM THANKFUL FOR ... 🙏
1._____
2._____
3._____

What did you eat today? 🍽

BREAKFAST	LUNCH	DINNER

SNACKS	Nutrition check list:

Nutrition check list:

4 Proteins [ ]   2 Fruits [ ]   Nuts [ ]
3 Veggies [ ]   2 Carb [ ]   Seeds [ ]

Water: 🥛🥛🥛🥛🥛🥛🥛🥛🥛🥛🥛

🧘 : [ ]   ⚖

SUPPLEMENTS/TABS 💊
_____
_____
_____
_____
_____

EXERCISE/YOGA/ACTIVITY 🏃
_____
_____
_____
_____
_____

SYMPTOMS/CRAVINGS/RESPONSE 🧍   ⚡ 🔋
_____
_____
_____

DATE: _____ CYCLE DAY : ☐ ⬦ MOOD: 😐😊😑😞😣

🌙 SLEPT FROM ___:___ TO ___:___ TOTAL HOURS : _____

I AM THANKFUL FOR ... 🙏
1._____
2._____
3._____

What did you eat today? 🍽

BREAKFAST	LUNCH	DINNER

SNACKS

Nutrition check list:

4 Proteins ☐   2 Fruits ☐   Nuts ☐
3 Veggies ☐   2 Carb ☐   Seeds ☐

Water: ☐☐☐☐☐☐☐☐☐☐☐

🧘 : ☐   ⚖ _____

SUPPLEMENTS/TABS 💊

_____
_____
_____
_____
_____

EXERCISE/YOGA/ACTIVITY 🏃

_____
_____
_____
_____
_____

SYMPTOMS/CRAVINGS/RESPONSE 🧍   ⚡ 🔋

_____
_____
_____

DATE: _____ CYCLE DAY : ☐ ◌ MOOD: 😀 🙂 😐 🙁 😣

🌙💤 SLEPT FROM ___:___ TO ___:___ TOTAL HOURS : _____

I AM THANKFUL FOR ... 🙏
1._____
2._____
3._____

What did you eat today? 🍽

BREAKFAST	LUNCH	DINNER

SNACKS	

Nutrition check list:

4 Proteins ☐	2 Fruits ☐	Nuts ☐
3 Veggies ☐	2 Carb ☐	Seeds ☐

Water: ⊔⊔⊔⊔⊔⊔⊔⊔⊔⊔⊔⊔

🧘 : ☐   ⏱ _____

SUPPLEMENTS/TABS 💊   EXERCISE/YOGA/ACTIVITY 🏃

_____   _____
_____   _____
_____   _____
_____   _____
_____   _____

SYMPTOMS/CRAVINGS/RESPONSE 🧍   ⚡ 🔋

_____
_____
_____

DATE: _____ CYCLE DAY : [ ] ⬦ MOOD: 😀 😊 😐 ☹️ 😣

🌙(z) SLEPT FROM ___:___ TO ___:___ TOTAL HOURS : _____

I AM THANKFUL FOR ... 🙏

1. _____
2. _____
3. _____

What did you eat today? 🍽️

BREAKFAST	LUNCH	DINNER

SNACKS	Nutrition check list:

Nutrition check list:

4 Proteins [ ]   2 Fruits [ ]   Nuts [ ]
3 Veggies [ ]   2 Carb [ ]   Seeds [ ]

Water: 🥛🥛🥛🥛🥛🥛🥛🥛🥛🥛🥛

🧘 : [ ]   ⚖️

SUPPLEMENTS/TABS 💊   EXERCISE/YOGA/ACTIVITY 🏃

_____   _____
_____   _____
_____   _____
_____   _____
_____   _____

SYMPTOMS/CRAVINGS/RESPONSE 🧍   ⚡ 🔋

_____
_____
_____

DATE: _____ CYCLE DAY : [ ] ⬡ MOOD: 😊 🙂 😐 🙁 ☹️

🌙💤 SLEPT FROM ___:___ TO ___:___ TOTAL HOURS : _____

I AM THANKFUL FOR ... 🙏

1. _____
2. _____
3. _____

What did you eat today? 🍽️

BREAKFAST	LUNCH	DINNER

SNACKS	**Nutrition check list:**

4 Proteins [ ]   2 Fruits [ ]   Nuts [ ]
3 Veggies [ ]   2 Carb [ ]   Seeds [ ]

Water: ⊔⊔⊔⊔⊔⊔⊔⊔⊔⊔⊔

🧘 : [ ]   ⚖️

SUPPLEMENTS/TABS 💊

EXERCISE/YOGA/ACTIVITY 🏃

_____   _____
_____   _____
_____   _____
_____   _____

SYMPTOMS/CRAVINGS/RESPONSE 🧍   ⚡ 🔋[ ][ ][ ]

_____
_____
_____

DATE: _____ CYCLE DAY : [   ] ⬡ MOOD: 😀 🙂 😐 🙁 😫

🌙💤 SLEPT FROM ___:___ TO ___:___   TOTAL HOURS : _____

I AM THANKFUL FOR ... 🙏

1._____
2._____
3._____

What did you eat today? 🍽️

BREAKFAST	LUNCH	DINNER

SNACKS

Nutrition check list:

| 4 Proteins | [   ] | 2 Fruits | [   ] | Nuts | [   ] |
| 3 Veggies | [   ] | 2 Carb | [   ] | Seeds | [   ] |

Water: 🥛🥛🥛🥛🥛🥛🥛🥛🥛🥛

🧘 : [   ]   ⚖️

SUPPLEMENTS/TABS 💊

EXERCISE/YOGA/ACTIVITY 🏃

_____   _____
_____   _____
_____   _____
_____   _____
_____   _____

SYMPTOMS/CRAVINGS/RESPONSE 🔍   ⚡ 🔋

_____
_____
_____

DATE: _____ CYCLE DAY : ☐ ⬡ MOOD: 😀 🙂 😐 ☹️ 😖

🌙 SLEPT FROM ___:___ TO ___:___ TOTAL HOURS : _____

I AM THANKFUL FOR ... 🙏

1._____
2._____
3._____

What did you eat today? 🍽️

BREAKFAST	LUNCH	DINNER

SNACKS	

Nutrition check list:

| 4 Proteins ☐ | 2 Fruits ☐ | Nuts ☐ |
| 3 Veggies ☐ | 2 Carb ☐ | Seeds ☐ |

Water: 🥛🥛🥛🥛🥛🥛🥛🥛🥛🥛🥛🥛

🧘 : ☐   ⚖️

SUPPLEMENTS/TABS 💊

_____
_____
_____
_____
_____

EXERCISE/YOGA/ACTIVITY 🏃

_____
_____
_____
_____
_____

SYMPTOMS/CRAVINGS/RESPONSE 🧍

⚡ 🔋

_____
_____
_____

DATE: _____ CYCLE DAY : [ ] ⬡ MOOD: 😀 🙂 😐 🙁 😣

🌙 SLEPT FROM ___:___ TO ___:___ TOTAL HOURS : _____

I AM THANKFUL FOR ... 🙏

1._____
2._____
3._____

What did you eat today? 🍽️

BREAKFAST	LUNCH	DINNER

SNACKS

Nutrition check list:

4 Proteins [ ]   2 Fruits [ ]   Nuts [ ]
3 Veggies [ ]   2 Carb [ ]   Seeds [ ]

Water: 🥛🥛🥛🥛🥛🥛🥛🥛🥛🥛

🧘 : [ ]   ⚖️

SUPPLEMENTS/TABS 💊

EXERCISE/YOGA/ACTIVITY 🏃

_____   _____
_____   _____
_____   _____
_____   _____
_____   _____

SYMPTOMS/CRAVINGS/RESPONSE 🧍   ⚡ 🔋

_____
_____
_____

DATE: _____   CYCLE DAY : ☐ ⬡   MOOD: 😀 🙂 😐 🙁 😣

🌙 SLEPT FROM ___:___ TO ___:___   TOTAL HOURS : _____

I AM THANKFUL FOR ... 🙏
1._____
2._____
3._____

What did you eat today? 🍽️

BREAKFAST	LUNCH	DINNER

SNACKS	Nutrition check list:

Nutrition check list:

| 4 Proteins ☐ | 2 Fruits ☐ | Nuts ☐ |
| 3 Veggies ☐ | 2 Carb ☐ | Seeds ☐ |

Water: 🥛🥛🥛🥛🥛🥛🥛🥛🥛🥛🥛

🧘 : ☐   ⏱️ ....

SUPPLEMENTS/TABS 💊   EXERCISE/YOGA/ACTIVITY 🏃

_____   _____
_____   _____
_____   _____
_____   _____

SYMPTOMS/CRAVINGS/RESPONSE 🧍   ⚡ 🔋

_____
_____
_____

DATE: _____ CYCLE DAY : [ ] ◇ MOOD: ☺ ☺ 😐 ☹ ☹

🌙 SLEPT FROM ___:___ TO ___:___ TOTAL HOURS : _____

I AM THANKFUL FOR ... 🙏

1. _____
2. _____
3. _____

What did you eat today? 🍽

BREAKFAST	LUNCH	DINNER

SNACKS

Nutrition check list:

4 Proteins [ ]   2 Fruits [ ]   Nuts [ ]
3 Veggies [ ]   2 Carb [ ]   Seeds [ ]

Water: ⊔⊔⊔⊔⊔⊔⊔⊔⊔⊔⊔

🧘 : [ ]   ⚖

SUPPLEMENTS/TABS 💊   EXERCISE/YOGA/ACTIVITY 🏃

_____   _____
_____   _____
_____   _____
_____   _____
_____   _____

SYMPTOMS/CRAVINGS/RESPONSE 🧍   ⚡ 🔋

_____
_____
_____

DATE: _____ CYCLE DAY : ☐ 💧 MOOD: 😀 🙂 😐 🙁 ☹️

🌙 SLEPT FROM ___:___ TO ___:___ TOTAL HOURS : _____

I AM THANKFUL FOR ... 🙏
1. _____
2. _____
3. _____

What did you eat today? 🍽️

BREAKFAST	LUNCH	DINNER

SNACKS

Nutrition check list:

4 Proteins ☐   2 Fruits ☐   Nuts ☐
3 Veggies ☐   2 Carb ☐   Seeds ☐

Water: 🥛🥛🥛🥛🥛🥛🥛🥛🥛🥛🥛

🧘 : ☐   ⚖️ ....

SUPPLEMENTS/TABS 💊   EXERCISE/YOGA/ACTIVITY 🏃

_____   _____
_____   _____
_____   _____
_____   _____

SYMPTOMS/CRAVINGS/RESPONSE 🧍   ⚡ 🔋

_____
_____
_____

DATE: _____ CYCLE DAY : [ ] ⬦ MOOD: 😐😊😑☹️😣

🌙 SLEPT FROM ___:___ TO ___:___ TOTAL HOURS : _____

I AM THANKFUL FOR ... 🙏

1._____
2._____
3._____

What did you eat today? 🍽️

BREAKFAST	LUNCH	DINNER

SNACKS

Nutrition check list:

4 Proteins [ ]   2 Fruits [ ]   Nuts [ ]
3 Veggies [ ]   2 Carb [ ]   Seeds [ ]

Water: 🥛🥛🥛🥛🥛🥛🥛🥛🥛🥛🥛

🧘 : [ ]   ⚖️

SUPPLEMENTS/TABS 💊   EXERCISE/YOGA/ACTIVITY 🏃

_____   _____
_____   _____
_____   _____
_____   _____

SYMPTOMS/CRAVINGS/RESPONSE 🧍   ⚡ 🔋

_____
_____
_____

DATE: _____ CYCLE DAY : ☐ ⬡ MOOD: 😀 🙂 😐 🙁 😣

🌙 SLEPT FROM ___:___ TO ___:___ TOTAL HOURS : _____

🙏 I AM THANKFUL FOR ...
1._____
2._____
3._____

What did you eat today? 🍽

BREAKFAST	LUNCH	DINNER

SNACKS

Nutrition check list:

4 Proteins ☐   2 Fruits ☐   Nuts ☐
3 Veggies ☐   2 Carb ☐   Seeds ☐

Water: 🥛🥛🥛🥛🥛🥛🥛🥛🥛🥛

🧘 : ☐   ⚖️

SUPPLEMENTS/TABS 💊
_____
_____
_____
_____
_____

EXERCISE/YOGA/ACTIVITY 🏃
_____
_____
_____
_____

SYMPTOMS/CRAVINGS/RESPONSE 🤹   ⚡ 🔋
_____
_____
_____

DATE: _____ CYCLE DAY: ☐ 💧 MOOD: 😊 🙂 😐 ☹️ 😣

🌙 SLEPT FROM ___:___ TO ___:___ TOTAL HOURS: _____

I AM THANKFUL FOR ... 🙏
1._____
2._____
3._____

What did you eat today? 🍽️

BREAKFAST	LUNCH	DINNER

SNACKS	Nutrition check list:

Nutrition check list:

4 Proteins ☐   2 Fruits ☐   Nuts ☐
3 Veggies ☐   2 Carb ☐   Seeds ☐

Water: 🥤🥤🥤🥤🥤🥤🥤🥤🥤🥤🥤🥤

🧘 : ☐   ⚖️ _____

SUPPLEMENTS/TABS 💊   EXERCISE/YOGA/ACTIVITY 🏃

_____   _____
_____   _____
_____   _____
_____   _____
_____   _____

SYMPTOMS/CRAVINGS/RESPONSE 🧍   ⚡ 🔋

_____
_____
_____

DATE: _____ CYCLE DAY : ☐ ⬦ MOOD: 😀 🙂 😐 🙁 😣

🌙 SLEPT FROM ___:___ TO ___:___ TOTAL HOURS : _____

I AM THANKFUL FOR ... 🙏
1._____
2._____
3._____

What did you eat today? 🍽

BREAKFAST	LUNCH	DINNER

SNACKS	Nutrition check list:

Nutrition check list:

4 Proteins ☐   2 Fruits ☐   Nuts ☐
3 Veggies ☐   2 Carb ☐   Seeds ☐

Water: 🥛🥛🥛🥛🥛🥛🥛🥛🥛🥛

🧘 : ☐   ⚖

SUPPLEMENTS/TABS 💊   EXERCISE/YOGA/ACTIVITY 🏃

_____   _____
_____   _____
_____   _____
_____   _____
_____   _____

SYMPTOMS/CRAVINGS/RESPONSE 🧍   ⚡ 🔋

_____
_____
_____

DATE: _____ CYCLE DAY : ☐ ⬠ MOOD: 😃 😊 😐 🙁 😣

🌙 SLEPT FROM ___:___ TO ___:___   TOTAL HOURS : _____

I AM THANKFUL FOR ... 🙏

1._____
2._____
3._____

What did you eat today? 🍽

BREAKFAST	LUNCH	DINNER

SNACKS	Nutrition check list:

Nutrition check list:

4 Proteins ☐   2 Fruits ☐   Nuts ☐
3 Veggies ☐   2 Carb ☐   Seeds ☐

Water: ⬛⬛⬛⬛⬛⬛⬛⬛⬛⬛⬛⬛

🧘 : ☐   ⚖

SUPPLEMENTS/TABS 💊   EXERCISE/YOGA/ACTIVITY 🏃

_____   _____
_____   _____
_____   _____
_____   _____
_____   _____

SYMPTOMS/CRAVINGS/RESPONSE 🧍   ⚡ 🔋

_____
_____
_____

DATE: _____ CYCLE DAY : [ ] 💧 MOOD: 😊 🙂 😐 🙁 😣

🌙💤 SLEPT FROM ___:___ TO ___:___ TOTAL HOURS : _____

I AM THANKFUL FOR ... 🙏
1._____
2._____
3._____

What did you eat today? 🍽

BREAKFAST	LUNCH	DINNER

SNACKS	Nutrition check list:

Nutrition check list:

4 Proteins [ ]   2 Fruits [ ]   Nuts [ ]
3 Veggies [ ]   2 Carb [ ]   Seeds [ ]

Water: 🥤🥤🥤🥤🥤🥤🥤🥤🥤🥤🥤🥤

🧘 : [ ]   ⚖

SUPPLEMENTS/TABS 💊   EXERCISE/YOGA/ACTIVITY 🏃

_____   _____
_____   _____
_____   _____
_____   _____

SYMPTOMS/CRAVINGS/RESPONSE 🧍   ⚡ 🔋

_____
_____
_____

DATE: _____ CYCLE DAY : ☐ ⬤ MOOD: 😀 🙂 😐 ☹️ 😫

🌙 SLEPT FROM ___:___ TO ___:___   TOTAL HOURS : _____

I AM THANKFUL FOR ... 🙏

1._____
2._____
3._____

What did you eat today? 🍽️

BREAKFAST	LUNCH	DINNER

SNACKS

Nutrition check list:

4 Proteins ☐   2 Fruits ☐   Nuts ☐
3 Veggies ☐   2 Carb ☐   Seeds ☐

Water: ⬛⬛⬛⬛⬛⬛⬛⬛⬛⬛⬛

🧘 : ☐   ⚖️ ....

SUPPLEMENTS/TABS 💊

EXERCISE/YOGA/ACTIVITY 🏃

_____   _____
_____   _____
_____   _____
_____   _____
_____   _____

SYMPTOMS/CRAVINGS/RESPONSE 🧍   ⚡ 🔋

_____
_____
_____

DATE: _____ CYCLE DAY : [   ] ◊ MOOD: 😃 🙂 😐 🙁 😫

🌙 SLEPT FROM ___:___ TO ___:___ TOTAL HOURS : _____

I AM THANKFUL FOR ... 🙏

1._____
2._____
3._____

What did you eat today? 🍽

BREAKFAST	LUNCH	DINNER

SNACKS

Nutrition check list:

4 Proteins [ ]   2 Fruits [ ]   Nuts [ ]
3 Veggies [ ]   2 Carb [ ]   Seeds [ ]

Water: 🥛🥛🥛🥛🥛🥛🥛🥛🥛🥛🥛

🧘 : [ ]   ⚖

SUPPLEMENTS/TABS 💊

_____
_____
_____
_____
_____

EXERCISE/YOGA/ACTIVITY 🏃

_____
_____
_____
_____

SYMPTOMS/CRAVINGS/RESPONSE 🧍

⚡ 🔋

_____
_____
_____

DATE: _____   CYCLE DAY : ☐ ⬡   MOOD: 😊😊😐☹️😣

🌙💤 SLEPT FROM ___:___ TO ___:___   TOTAL HOURS : _____

I AM THANKFUL FOR ... 🙏
1._____
2._____
3._____

What did you eat today? 🍽️

BREAKFAST	LUNCH	DINNER

SNACKS	Nutrition check list:

Nutrition check list:
4 Proteins ☐   2 Fruits ☐   Nuts ☐
3 Veggies ☐   2 Carb ☐   Seeds ☐

Water: 🥛🥛🥛🥛🥛🥛🥛🥛🥛🥛🥛🥛

🧘 : ☐   ⚖️ ....

SUPPLEMENTS/TABS 💊
_____
_____
_____
_____
_____

EXERCISE/YOGA/ACTIVITY 🏃
_____
_____
_____
_____

SYMPTOMS/CRAVINGS/RESPONSE 🧍   ⚡ 🔋
_____
_____
_____

DATE: _____ CYCLE DAY : ☐ ⬡ MOOD: 😊 🙂 😐 🙁 😣

🌙💤 SLEPT FROM ___:___ TO ___:___ TOTAL HOURS : _____

I AM THANKFUL FOR ... 🙏
1._____
2._____
3._____

What did you eat today? 🍽

BREAKFAST	LUNCH	DINNER

SNACKS	Nutrition check list:

Nutrition check list:

4 Proteins ☐   2 Fruits ☐   Nuts ☐
3 Veggies ☐   2 Carb ☐   Seeds ☐

Water: 🥛🥛🥛🥛🥛🥛🥛🥛🥛🥛🥛

🧘 : ☐   ⚖ _____

SUPPLEMENTS/TABS 💊   EXERCISE/YOGA/ACTIVITY 🏃

_____   _____
_____   _____
_____   _____
_____   _____
_____   _____

SYMPTOMS/CRAVINGS/RESPONSE 🧍   ⚡ 🔋

_____
_____
_____

DATE: _____ CYCLE DAY : ☐ 💧 MOOD: 😃 🙂 😐 🙁 😫

🌙💤 SLEPT FROM ___:___ TO ___:___   TOTAL HOURS : _____

I AM THANKFUL FOR ... 🙏

1._____
2._____
3._____

What did you eat today? 🍽️

BREAKFAST	LUNCH	DINNER

SNACKS	Nutrition check list:

Nutrition check list:

4 Proteins ☐   2 Fruits ☐   Nuts ☐
3 Veggies ☐   2 Carb ☐   Seeds ☐

Water: 🥛🥛🥛🥛🥛🥛🥛🥛🥛🥛

🧘 : ☐   ⚖️

SUPPLEMENTS/TABS 💊   EXERCISE/YOGA/ACTIVITY 🏃

_____   _____
_____   _____
_____   _____
_____   _____
_____   _____

SYMPTOMS/CRAVINGS/RESPONSE 🧍   ⚡ 🔋

_____
_____
_____

DATE: _____   CYCLE DAY : ☐ 💧   MOOD: 😊 🙂 😐 🙁 😣

🌙💤 SLEPT FROM ___:___ TO ___:___   TOTAL HOURS : _____

I AM THANKFUL FOR ... 🙏
1. _____
2. _____
3. _____

What did you eat today? 🍽

BREAKFAST	LUNCH	DINNER

SNACKS

Nutrition check list:

4 Proteins ☐   2 Fruits ☐   Nuts ☐
3 Veggies ☐   2 Carb ☐   Seeds ☐

Water: 🥛🥛🥛🥛🥛🥛🥛🥛🥛🥛

🧘 : ☐   ⚖️

SUPPLEMENTS/TABS 💊

_____
_____
_____
_____

EXERCISE/YOGA/ACTIVITY 🏃

_____
_____
_____
_____

SYMPTOMS/CRAVINGS/RESPONSE 🧍   ⚡ 🔋

_____
_____
_____

DATE: _____ CYCLE DAY : ☐ ⬡ MOOD: 😀 🙂 😐 😟 😫

🌙 SLEPT FROM ___:___ TO ___:___ TOTAL HOURS : _____

I AM THANKFUL FOR ... 🙏

1._____
2._____
3._____

What did you eat today? 🍽️

BREAKFAST	LUNCH	DINNER

SNACKS

Nutrition check list:

4 Proteins ☐   2 Fruits ☐   Nuts ☐
3 Veggies ☐   2 Carb ☐   Seeds ☐

Water: 🥛🥛🥛🥛🥛🥛🥛🥛🥛🥛

🧘 : ☐   ⚖️ _____

SUPPLEMENTS/TABS 💊   EXERCISE/YOGA/ACTIVITY 🏃

_____   _____
_____   _____
_____   _____
_____   _____
_____   _____

SYMPTOMS/CRAVINGS/RESPONSE 🧍   ⚡ 🔋

_____
_____
_____

DATE: _____ CYCLE DAY : ☐ 🌢 MOOD: 😃 🙂 😐 🙁 😣

🌙💤 SLEPT FROM ___:___ TO ___:___   TOTAL HOURS : _____

I AM THANKFUL FOR ... 🙏
1._____
2._____
3._____

What did you eat today? 🍽

BREAKFAST	LUNCH	DINNER

SNACKS

Nutrition check list:

4 Proteins ☐   2 Fruits ☐   Nuts ☐
3 Veggies ☐   2 Carb ☐   Seeds ☐

Water: 🥛🥛🥛🥛🥛🥛🥛🥛🥛🥛🥛

🧘 : ☐   ⚖

SUPPLEMENTS/TABS 💊

_____
_____
_____
_____
_____

EXERCISE/YOGA/ACTIVITY 🏃

_____
_____
_____
_____
_____

SYMPTOMS/CRAVINGS/RESPONSE 🧖   ⚡ 🔋

_____
_____
_____

DATE: _____   CYCLE DAY : [　]◇   MOOD: 😃😊😐😟😣

🌙 SLEPT FROM ___:___ TO ___:___   TOTAL HOURS : _____

I AM THANKFUL FOR ... 🙏
1._____
2._____
3._____

What did you eat today? 🍽

BREAKFAST	LUNCH	DINNER

SNACKS	Nutrition check list:
	4 Proteins [　] 2 Fruits [　] Nuts [　]
	3 Veggies [　] 2 Carb [　] Seeds [　]

Water: ⊔⊔⊔⊔⊔⊔⊔⊔⊔⊔⊔⊔

🧘 : [　]   ⚖ _____

SUPPLEMENTS/TABS 💊   EXERCISE/YOGA/ACTIVITY 🏃

_____   _____
_____   _____
_____   _____
_____   _____
_____   _____

SYMPTOMS/CRAVINGS/RESPONSE 🧍   ⚡ 🔋

_____
_____
_____

DATE: _____ CYCLE DAY : ☐ ⬡ MOOD: 😀 🙂 😐 🙁 ☹️

🌙 SLEPT FROM ___:___ TO ___:___ TOTAL HOURS : _____

I AM THANKFUL FOR ... 🙏

1._____
2._____
3._____

What did you eat today? 🍽️

BREAKFAST	LUNCH	DINNER

SNACKS	Nutrition check list:

Nutrition check list:

4 Proteins ☐   2 Fruits ☐   Nuts ☐
3 Veggies ☐   2 Carb ☐   Seeds ☐

Water: 🥤🥤🥤🥤🥤🥤🥤🥤🥤🥤🥤

🧘 : ☐   ⚖️ _____

SUPPLEMENTS/TABS 💊   EXERCISE/YOGA/ACTIVITY 🏃

_____   _____
_____   _____
_____   _____
_____   _____
_____   _____

SYMPTOMS/CRAVINGS/RESPONSE 🧍   ⚡ 🔋

_____
_____
_____

DATE: _____ CYCLE DAY : ☐ ⬦ MOOD: 😀 🙂 😐 🙁 😣

🌙 SLEPT FROM ___:___ TO ___:___ TOTAL HOURS : _____

I AM THANKFUL FOR ... 🙏
1._____
2._____
3._____

What did you eat today? 🍽

BREAKFAST	LUNCH	DINNER

SNACKS

Nutrition check list:

4 Proteins ☐   2 Fruits ☐   Nuts ☐
3 Veggies ☐   2 Carb ☐   Seeds ☐

Water: ⬜⬜⬜⬜⬜⬜⬜⬜⬜⬜⬜

🧘 : ☐   ⚖ _____

SUPPLEMENTS/TABS 💊

EXERCISE/YOGA/ACTIVITY 🏃

_____   _____
_____   _____
_____   _____
_____   _____
_____   _____

SYMPTOMS/CRAVINGS/RESPONSE 🧍   ⚡ 🔋

_____
_____
_____

DATE: _____ CYCLE DAY : ☐ ⬡ MOOD: 😊 🙂 😐 🙁 😣

🌙 SLEPT FROM ___:___ TO ___:___ TOTAL HOURS : _____

I AM THANKFUL FOR ... 🙏

1._____
2._____
3._____

What did you eat today? 🍽️

BREAKFAST	LUNCH	DINNER

SNACKS

Nutrition check list:

4 Proteins ☐   2 Fruits ☐   Nuts ☐
3 Veggies ☐   2 Carb ☐   Seeds ☐

Water: 🥤🥤🥤🥤🥤🥤🥤🥤🥤🥤🥤

🧘 : ☐   ⚖️ _____

SUPPLEMENTS/TABS 💊   EXERCISE/YOGA/ACTIVITY 🏃

_____   _____
_____   _____
_____   _____
_____   _____
_____   _____

SYMPTOMS/CRAVINGS/RESPONSE 🧍   ⚡ 🔋

_____
_____
_____

DATE: _____   CYCLE DAY : [ ] ⬙   MOOD: 😀 ☺ 😐 ☹ 😣

🌙 SLEPT FROM ___:___ TO ___:___   TOTAL HOURS : _____

I AM THANKFUL FOR ... 🙏

1._____

2._____

3._____

What did you eat today? 🍽

BREAKFAST	LUNCH	DINNER

SNACKS	Nutrition check list:

Nutrition check list:

4 Proteins [ ]   2 Fruits [ ]   Nuts [ ]
3 Veggies [ ]   2 Carb [ ]   Seeds [ ]

Water: 🥛🥛🥛🥛🥛🥛🥛🥛🥛🥛

🧘 : [ ]   ⚖ _____

SUPPLEMENTS/TABS 💊

_____
_____
_____
_____
_____

EXERCISE/YOGA/ACTIVITY 🏃

_____
_____
_____
_____
_____

SYMPTOMS/CRAVINGS/RESPONSE 🧍   ⚡ 🔋

_____
_____
_____

DATE: _____ CYCLE DAY : [ ] ⬡ MOOD: 😀 ☺ 😐 ☹ 😣

🌙 SLEPT FROM ___:___ TO ___:___ TOTAL HOURS : _____

I AM THANKFUL FOR ... 🙏

1._____
2._____
3._____

What did you eat today? 🍽

BREAKFAST	LUNCH	DINNER

SNACKS

Nutrition check list:

4 Proteins [ ]   2 Fruits [ ]   Nuts [ ]
3 Veggies [ ]   2 Carb [ ]   Seeds [ ]

Water: 🥛🥛🥛🥛🥛🥛🥛🥛🥛🥛🥛

🧘 : [ ]   ⚖

SUPPLEMENTS/TABS 💊   EXERCISE/YOGA/ACTIVITY 🏃

_____   _____
_____   _____
_____   _____
_____   _____
_____   _____

SYMPTOMS/CRAVINGS/RESPONSE 🧍   ⚡ 🔋

_____
_____
_____

DATE: _____   CYCLE DAY : ☐ ⬦   MOOD: 😊 🙂 😐 🙁 😣

🌙💤 SLEPT FROM ___:___ TO ___:___   TOTAL HOURS : _____

I AM THANKFUL FOR ... 🙏
1._____
2._____
3._____

What did you eat today? 🍽️

BREAKFAST	LUNCH	DINNER

SNACKS	Nutrition check list:

Nutrition check list:

4 Proteins ☐   2 Fruits ☐   Nuts ☐
3 Veggies ☐   2 Carb ☐   Seeds ☐

Water: 🥛🥛🥛🥛🥛🥛🥛🥛🥛🥛🥛

🧘 : ☐   ⚖️ ....

SUPPLEMENTS/TABS 💊   EXERCISE/YOGA/ACTIVITY 🏃

_____   _____
_____   _____
_____   _____
_____   _____
_____   _____

SYMPTOMS/CRAVINGS/RESPONSE 🧍   ⚡ 🔋

_____
_____
_____

DATE: _____ CYCLE DAY : ☐ ◯ MOOD: 😀 🙂 😐 🙁 😫

🌙 SLEPT FROM ___:___ TO ___:___ TOTAL HOURS : _____

I AM THANKFUL FOR ... 🙏
1._____
2._____
3._____

What did you eat today? 🍽

BREAKFAST	LUNCH	DINNER

SNACKS	Nutrition check list:

Nutrition check list:

4 Proteins ☐   2 Fruits ☐   Nuts ☐
3 Veggies ☐   2 Carb ☐   Seeds ☐

Water: 🥛🥛🥛🥛🥛🥛🥛🥛🥛🥛

🧘 : ☐   ⚖

SUPPLEMENTS/TABS 💊

_____
_____
_____
_____

EXERCISE/YOGA/ACTIVITY 🏃

_____
_____
_____
_____

SYMPTOMS/CRAVINGS/RESPONSE 🧍   ⚡ 🔋

_____
_____
_____

DATE: _____ CYCLE DAY : [ ] ⬡ MOOD: 😀 🙂 😐 🙁 😣

🌙💤 SLEPT FROM ___:___ TO ___:___   TOTAL HOURS : _____

I AM THANKFUL FOR ... 🙏

1._____
2._____
3._____

What did you eat today? 🍽

BREAKFAST	LUNCH	DINNER

SNACKS

Nutrition check list:

4 Proteins	[ ]	2 Fruits	[ ]	Nuts	[ ]
3 Veggies	[ ]	2 Carb	[ ]	Seeds	[ ]

Water: 🥛🥛🥛🥛🥛🥛🥛🥛🥛🥛🥛

🧘 : [ ]   ⚖ ....

SUPPLEMENTS/TABS 💊

EXERCISE/YOGA/ACTIVITY 🏃

_____   _____
_____   _____
_____   _____
_____   _____

SYMPTOMS/CRAVINGS/RESPONSE 🧍   ⚡ 🔋

_____
_____
_____

DATE: _____ CYCLE DAY : ☐ ⬡ MOOD: 😄 🙂 😐 🙁 😣

🌙💤 SLEPT FROM ___:___ TO ___:___ TOTAL HOURS : _____

I AM THANKFUL FOR ... 🙏

1. _____
2. _____
3. _____

What did you eat today? 🍽️

BREAKFAST	LUNCH	DINNER

SNACKS

Nutrition check list:

4 Proteins ☐   2 Fruits ☐   Nuts ☐
3 Veggies ☐   2 Carb ☐   Seeds ☐

Water: 🥛🥛🥛🥛🥛🥛🥛🥛🥛🥛

🧘 : ☐   ⏲️

SUPPLEMENTS/TABS 💊

_____
_____
_____
_____

EXERCISE/YOGA/ACTIVITY 🏃

_____
_____
_____
_____

SYMPTOMS/CRAVINGS/RESPONSE 🧍   ⚡ 🔋

_____
_____
_____

DATE: _____ CYCLE DAY : ☐ ⬡ MOOD: 😃 🙂 😐 🙁 ☹️

🌙 SLEPT FROM ___:___ TO ___:___ TOTAL HOURS : _____

I AM THANKFUL FOR ... 🙏
1._____
2._____
3._____

What did you eat today? 🍽️

BREAKFAST	LUNCH	DINNER

SNACKS

Nutrition check list:

4 Proteins ☐   2 Fruits ☐   Nuts ☐
3 Veggies ☐   2 Carb ☐   Seeds ☐

Water: 🥛🥛🥛🥛🥛🥛🥛🥛🥛🥛🥛

🧘 : ☐   ⚖️ _____

SUPPLEMENTS/TABS 💊   EXERCISE/YOGA/ACTIVITY 🏃

_____   _____
_____   _____
_____   _____
_____   _____

SYMPTOMS/CRAVINGS/RESPONSE 🧍   ⚡ 🔋

_____
_____
_____

DATE: _____   CYCLE DAY : ☐ ⬦   MOOD: 😄 🙂 😐 🙁 😣

🌙 SLEPT FROM ___:___ TO ___:___   TOTAL HOURS : _____

I AM THANKFUL FOR ... 🙏
1._____
2._____
3._____

What did you eat today? 🍽

BREAKFAST	LUNCH	DINNER

SNACKS	**Nutrition check list:**

4 Proteins ☐   2 Fruits ☐   Nuts ☐
3 Veggies ☐   2 Carb ☐   Seeds ☐

Water: 🥛🥛🥛🥛🥛🥛🥛🥛🥛🥛

🧘 : ☐   ⚖

SUPPLEMENTS/TABS 💊   EXERCISE/YOGA/ACTIVITY 🏃
_____   _____
_____   _____
_____   _____
_____   _____
_____   _____

SYMPTOMS/CRAVINGS/RESPONSE 🧘   ⚡ 🔋
_____
_____
_____

DATE: _____   CYCLE DAY : [   ] ⬦   MOOD: 😀 🙂 😐 🙁 😣

🌙💤 SLEPT FROM ___:___ TO ___:___   TOTAL HOURS : _____

I AM THANKFUL FOR ... 🙏

1._____
2._____
3._____

What did you eat today? 🍽

BREAKFAST	LUNCH	DINNER

SNACKS	Nutrition check list:

Nutrition check list:

4 Proteins [ ]   2 Fruits [ ]   Nuts [ ]
3 Veggies [ ]   2 Carb [ ]   Seeds [ ]

Water: 🥛🥛🥛🥛🥛🥛🥛🥛🥛🥛🥛🥛

🧘 : [ ]   ⚖

SUPPLEMENTS/TABS 💊

_____
_____
_____
_____
_____

EXERCISE/YOGA/ACTIVITY 🏃

_____
_____
_____
_____

SYMPTOMS/CRAVINGS/RESPONSE 🧍

⚡ 🔋

_____
_____
_____

DATE: _____ CYCLE DAY : [ ] ⬡ MOOD: 😊 🙂 😐 🙁 ☹️

🌙💤 SLEPT FROM ___:___ TO ___:___ TOTAL HOURS : _____

I AM THANKFUL FOR ... 🙏

1._____
2._____
3._____

What did you eat today? 🍽️

BREAKFAST	LUNCH	DINNER

SNACKS	Nutrition check list:

Nutrition check list:

4 Proteins [ ]	2 Fruits [ ]	Nuts [ ]
3 Veggies [ ]	2 Carb [ ]	Seeds [ ]

Water: ▯▯▯▯▯▯▯▯▯▯▯▯

🧘 : [ ]   ⚖️ _____

SUPPLEMENTS/TABS 💊   EXERCISE/YOGA/ACTIVITY 🏃

_____   _____
_____   _____
_____   _____
_____   _____
_____   _____

SYMPTOMS/CRAVINGS/RESPONSE 🧍   ⚡ 🔋

_____
_____
_____

DATE: _____ CYCLE DAY : ☐ ◯ MOOD: 😀 🙂 😐 ☹️ 😫

🌙 SLEPT FROM ___:___ TO ___:___ TOTAL HOURS : _____

I AM THANKFUL FOR ... 🙏

1. _____
2. _____
3. _____

What did you eat today? 🍽️

BREAKFAST	LUNCH	DINNER

SNACKS	Nutrition check list:

Nutrition check list:

4 Proteins ☐   2 Fruits ☐   Nuts ☐
3 Veggies ☐   2 Carb ☐   Seeds ☐

Water: 🥛🥛🥛🥛🥛🥛🥛🥛🥛🥛🥛

🧘 : ☐   ⚖️ _____

SUPPLEMENTS/TABS 💊

EXERCISE/YOGA/ACTIVITY 🏃

_____   _____
_____   _____
_____   _____
_____   _____
_____   _____

SYMPTOMS/CRAVINGS/RESPONSE 🧍   ⚡ 🔋

_____
_____
_____

DATE: _____ CYCLE DAY : [ ] ⬦ MOOD: 😊 🙂 😐 ☹️ 😣

🌙 SLEPT FROM ___:___ TO ___:___ TOTAL HOURS : _____

I AM THANKFUL FOR ... 🙏
1._____
2._____
3._____

What did you eat today? 🍽️

BREAKFAST	LUNCH	DINNER

SNACKS

Nutrition check list:

4 Proteins [ ]   2 Fruits [ ]   Nuts [ ]
3 Veggies [ ]   2 Carb [ ]   Seeds [ ]

Water: 🥛🥛🥛🥛🥛🥛🥛🥛🥛🥛

🧘 : [ ]   ⚖️

SUPPLEMENTS/TABS 💊   EXERCISE/YOGA/ACTIVITY 🏃

_____   _____
_____   _____
_____   _____
_____   _____
_____   _____

SYMPTOMS/CRAVINGS/RESPONSE 🧍   ⚡ [▯▯▯]

_____
_____
_____

DATE: _____ CYCLE DAY : [ ] ⬦ MOOD: 😜 🙂 😐 🙁 😣

🌙 SLEPT FROM ___:___ TO ___:___ TOTAL HOURS : _____

I AM THANKFUL FOR ... 🙏

1._____
2._____
3._____

What did you eat today? 🍽

BREAKFAST	LUNCH	DINNER

SNACKS

Nutrition check list:

4 Proteins [ ]   2 Fruits [ ]   Nuts [ ]
3 Veggies [ ]   2 Carb [ ]   Seeds [ ]

Water: 🥛🥛🥛🥛🥛🥛🥛🥛🥛🥛🥛

🧘 : [ ]   ⚖

SUPPLEMENTS/TABS 💊   EXERCISE/YOGA/ACTIVITY 🏃

_____   _____
_____   _____
_____   _____
_____   _____

SYMPTOMS/CRAVINGS/RESPONSE 🧍   ⚡ 🔋

_____
_____
_____

DATE: _____ CYCLE DAY : ☐ ⬤ MOOD: 😀 🙂 😐 🙁 😣

🌙💤 SLEPT FROM ___:___ TO ___:___ TOTAL HOURS : _____

I AM THANKFUL FOR ... 🙏
1._____
2._____
3._____

What did you eat today? 🍽️

BREAKFAST	LUNCH	DINNER

SNACKS	Nutrition check list:

Nutrition check list:

4 Proteins ☐   2 Fruits ☐   Nuts ☐
3 Veggies ☐   2 Carb ☐   Seeds ☐

Water: 🥛🥛🥛🥛🥛🥛🥛🥛🥛🥛🥛🥛

🧘 : ☐   ⚖️ ....

SUPPLEMENTS/TABS 💊   EXERCISE/YOGA/ACTIVITY 🏃
_____   _____
_____   _____
_____   _____
_____   _____
_____   _____

SYMPTOMS/CRAVINGS/RESPONSE 🧘   ⚡ 🔋
_____
_____
_____

DATE: _____ CYCLE DAY : [ ] ⬦ MOOD: 😃 🙂 😐 🙁 😣

🌙 SLEPT FROM ___:___ TO ___:___ TOTAL HOURS : _____

I AM THANKFUL FOR ... 🙏
1._____
2._____
3._____

What did you eat today? 🍽

BREAKFAST	LUNCH	DINNER

SNACKS	**Nutrition check list:**

Nutrition check list:

4 Proteins	[ ]	2 Fruits	[ ]	Nuts	[ ]
3 Veggies	[ ]	2 Carb	[ ]	Seeds	[ ]

Water: ⊔⊔⊔⊔⊔⊔⊔⊔⊔⊔⊔

🧘 : [ ]   ⚖ _____

SUPPLEMENTS/TABS 💊   EXERCISE/YOGA/ACTIVITY 🏃

_____   _____
_____   _____
_____   _____
_____   _____
_____   _____

SYMPTOMS/CRAVINGS/RESPONSE 🧍   ⚡ 🔋

_____
_____
_____

DATE: _____   CYCLE DAY : [ ] ⬭ MOOD: 😐 🙂 😐 ☹️ 😫

🌙 z z SLEPT FROM ___:___ TO ___:___   TOTAL HOURS : _____

I AM THANKFUL FOR ... 🙏
1._____
2._____
3._____

What did you eat today? 🍽️

BREAKFAST	LUNCH	DINNER

SNACKS	Nutrition check list:

Nutrition check list:

4 Proteins [ ]   2 Fruits [ ]   Nuts [ ]
3 Veggies [ ]   2 Carb [ ]   Seeds [ ]

Water: 🥛🥛🥛🥛🥛🥛🥛🥛🥛🥛🥛

🧘 : [ ]   ⚖️ _____

SUPPLEMENTS/TABS 💊   EXERCISE/YOGA/ACTIVITY 🏃

_____   _____
_____   _____
_____   _____
_____   _____
_____   _____

SYMPTOMS/CRAVINGS/RESPONSE 🧍   ⚡ 🔋

_____
_____
_____

DATE: _____ CYCLE DAY : ☐ 💧 MOOD: 😀 🙂 😐 🙁 😣

🌙💤 SLEPT FROM ___:___ TO ___:___ TOTAL HOURS : _____

I AM THANKFUL FOR ... 🙏

1. _____
2. _____
3. _____

What did you eat today? 🍽️

BREAKFAST	LUNCH	DINNER

| SNACKS | Nutrition check list: |

Nutrition check list:

4 Proteins ☐   2 Fruits ☐   Nuts ☐
3 Veggies ☐   2 Carb ☐   Seeds ☐

Water: 🥤🥤🥤🥤🥤🥤🥤🥤🥤🥤

🧘 : ☐   ⚖️

SUPPLEMENTS/TABS 💊

_____
_____
_____
_____
_____

EXERCISE/YOGA/ACTIVITY 🏃

_____
_____
_____
_____

SYMPTOMS/CRAVINGS/RESPONSE 🔍   ⚡ 🔋

_____
_____
_____

DATE: _____ CYCLE DAY : ☐ ⬡ MOOD: 😀 🙂 😐 🙁 😣

🌙💤 SLEPT FROM ___:___ TO ___:___ TOTAL HOURS : _____

I AM THANKFUL FOR ... 🙏
1._____
2._____
3._____

What did you eat today? 🍽️

BREAKFAST	LUNCH	DINNER

SNACKS	Nutrition check list:
	4 Proteins ☐ 2 Fruits ☐ Nuts ☐
	3 Veggies ☐ 2 Carb ☐ Seeds ☐

Water: 🥛🥛🥛🥛🥛🥛🥛🥛🥛🥛🥛

🧘 : ☐   ⏲️

SUPPLEMENTS/TABS 💊   EXERCISE/YOGA/ACTIVITY 🏃

_____   _____
_____   _____
_____   _____
_____   _____

SYMPTOMS/CRAVINGS/RESPONSE 🧍   ⚡ 🔋

_____
_____
_____

DATE: _____ CYCLE DAY : ☐ ◊ MOOD: 😃 🙂 😐 🙁 😫

🌙 SLEPT FROM ___:___ TO ___:___ TOTAL HOURS : _____

I AM THANKFUL FOR ... 🙏

1. _____
2. _____
3. _____

What did you eat today? 🍽

BREAKFAST	LUNCH	DINNER

SNACKS

Nutrition check list:

| 4 Proteins ☐ | 2 Fruits ☐ | Nuts ☐ |
| 3 Veggies ☐ | 2 Carb ☐ | Seeds ☐ |

Water: 🥛🥛🥛🥛🥛🥛🥛🥛🥛🥛

🧘 : ☐   ⚖️

SUPPLEMENTS/TABS 💊

_____
_____
_____
_____
_____

EXERCISE/YOGA/ACTIVITY 🏃

_____
_____
_____
_____
_____

SYMPTOMS/CRAVINGS/RESPONSE 🔍   ⚡ 🔋

_____
_____
_____

DATE: _____ CYCLE DAY : [ ] ◌ MOOD: 😃 🙂 😐 🙁 😫

🌙 SLEPT FROM ___:___ TO ___:___ TOTAL HOURS : _____

I AM THANKFUL FOR ... 🙏
1._____
2._____
3._____

What did you eat today? 🍽️

BREAKFAST	LUNCH	DINNER

SNACKS	Nutrition check list:

Nutrition check list:

4 Proteins [ ]   2 Fruits [ ]   Nuts [ ]
3 Veggies [ ]   2 Carb [ ]   Seeds [ ]

Water: 🥛🥛🥛🥛🥛🥛🥛🥛🥛🥛🥛

🧘 : [ ]   ⚖️ _____

SUPPLEMENTS/TABS 💊

_____
_____
_____
_____
_____

EXERCISE/YOGA/ACTIVITY 🏃

_____
_____
_____
_____
_____

SYMPTOMS/CRAVINGS/RESPONSE 🧍   ⚡ 🔋

_____
_____
_____

DATE: _____ CYCLE DAY : ☐ ⬤ MOOD: 😀 🙂 😐 🙁 😣

🌙💤 SLEPT FROM ___:___ TO ___:___ TOTAL HOURS : _____

I AM THANKFUL FOR ... 🙏

1. _____

2. _____

3. _____

What did you eat today? 🍽

BREAKFAST	LUNCH	DINNER

SNACKS	Nutrition check list:
	4 Proteins ☐ 2 Fruits ☐ Nuts ☐
	3 Veggies ☐ 2 Carb ☐ Seeds ☐

Water: 🥤🥤🥤🥤🥤🥤🥤🥤🥤🥤🥤

🧘 : ☐   ⚖ _____

SUPPLEMENTS/TABS 💊

_____   EXERCISE/YOGA/ACTIVITY 🏃

_____   _____

_____   _____

_____   _____

_____   _____

SYMPTOMS/CRAVINGS/RESPONSE 🧍   ⚡ 🔋

_____

_____

_____

DATE: _____   CYCLE DAY : [ ] ◊ MOOD: ☺ ☺ 😐 ☹ ☹

🌙 SLEPT FROM ___:___ TO ___:___   TOTAL HOURS : _____

I AM THANKFUL FOR ... 🙏
1._____
2._____
3._____

What did you eat today? 🍽

BREAKFAST	LUNCH	DINNER

SNACKS

Nutrition check list:
4 Proteins [ ]   2 Fruits [ ]   Nuts [ ]
3 Veggies [ ]   2 Carb [ ]   Seeds [ ]

Water: ⊔⊔⊔⊔⊔⊔⊔⊔⊔⊔⊔⊔

🧘 : [ ]   ⚖

SUPPLEMENTS/TABS 💊   EXERCISE/YOGA/ACTIVITY 🏃

_____   _____
_____   _____
_____   _____
_____   _____
_____   _____

SYMPTOMS/CRAVINGS/RESPONSE 🧍   ⚡ 🔋

_____
_____
_____

DATE: _____ CYCLE DAY : ☐ 💧 MOOD: 😃 🙂 😐 🙁 😣

🌙 SLEPT FROM ___:___ TO ___:___ TOTAL HOURS : _____

I AM THANKFUL FOR ... 🙏

1. _____
2. _____
3. _____

What did you eat today? 🍽️

BREAKFAST	LUNCH	DINNER

SNACKS

Nutrition check list:

4 Proteins ☐   2 Fruits ☐   Nuts ☐
3 Veggies ☐   2 Carb ☐   Seeds ☐

Water: 🥛🥛🥛🥛🥛🥛🥛🥛🥛🥛

🧘 : ☐   ⚖️ ....

SUPPLEMENTS/TABS 💊   EXERCISE/YOGA/ACTIVITY 🏃

_____   _____
_____   _____
_____   _____
_____   _____

_____   _____

SYMPTOMS/CRAVINGS/RESPONSE 🧍   ⚡ 🔋

_____
_____
_____

DATE: _____ CYCLE DAY : [ ] 🜄 MOOD: 😀 🙂 😐 🙁 😣

🌙 SLEPT FROM ___:___ TO ___:___ TOTAL HOURS : _____

I AM THANKFUL FOR ... 🙏
1._____
2._____
3._____

What did you eat today? 🍽

BREAKFAST	LUNCH	DINNER

SNACKS

Nutrition check list:

4 Proteins [ ] 2 Fruits [ ] Nuts [ ]
3 Veggies [ ] 2 Carb [ ] Seeds [ ]

Water: ▭▭▭▭▭▭▭▭▭▭▭

🧘 : [ ] ⚖

SUPPLEMENTS/TABS 💊

EXERCISE/YOGA/ACTIVITY 🏃

_____ _____
_____ _____
_____ _____
_____ _____

SYMPTOMS/CRAVINGS/RESPONSE 🧍 ⚡ 🔋

_____
_____
_____

DATE: _____ CYCLE DAY : ☐ ◇ MOOD: 😃 🙂 😐 ☹️ 😣

🌙💤 SLEPT FROM ___:___ TO ___:___ TOTAL HOURS : _____

I AM THANKFUL FOR ... 🙏
1._____
2._____
3._____

What did you eat today? 🍽️

BREAKFAST	LUNCH	DINNER

SNACKS

Nutrition check list:

4 Proteins ☐   2 Fruits ☐   Nuts ☐
3 Veggies ☐   2 Carb ☐   Seeds ☐

Water: ⬜⬜⬜⬜⬜⬜⬜⬜⬜⬜

🧘 : ☐   ⚖️ _____

SUPPLEMENTS/TABS 💊   EXERCISE/YOGA/ACTIVITY 🏃

_____   _____
_____   _____
_____   _____
_____   _____

SYMPTOMS/CRAVINGS/RESPONSE 🧍   ⚡ 🔋

_____
_____
_____

DATE: _____ CYCLE DAY : [ ] ⬦ MOOD: 😃 🙂 😐 🙁 😫

🌙 SLEPT FROM ___:___ TO ___:___ TOTAL HOURS : _____

I AM THANKFUL FOR ... 🙏
1._____
2._____
3._____

What did you eat today? 🍽

BREAKFAST	LUNCH	DINNER

SNACKS	Nutrition check list:

Nutrition check list:

4 Proteins [ ]   2 Fruits [ ]   Nuts [ ]
3 Veggies [ ]   2 Carb [ ]   Seeds [ ]

Water: 🥛🥛🥛🥛🥛🥛🥛🥛🥛🥛🥛

🧘 : [ ]   ⚖

SUPPLEMENTS/TABS 💊   EXERCISE/YOGA/ACTIVITY 🏃

_____   _____
_____   _____
_____   _____
_____   _____
_____   _____

SYMPTOMS/CRAVINGS/RESPONSE 🧍   ⚡ 🔋

_____
_____
_____

DATE: _____ CYCLE DAY : [ ] ◯ MOOD: 😃 🙂 😐 🙁 😣

🌙💤 SLEPT FROM ___:___ TO ___:___ TOTAL HOURS : _____

I AM THANKFUL FOR ... 🙏

1._____
2._____
3._____

What did you eat today? 🍽

BREAKFAST	LUNCH	DINNER

SNACKS	Nutrition check list:

Nutrition check list:

4 Proteins [ ]   2 Fruits [ ]   Nuts [ ]
3 Veggies [ ]   2 Carb [ ]   Seeds [ ]

Water: ⎕⎕⎕⎕⎕⎕⎕⎕⎕⎕

🧘 : [ ]   ⚖

SUPPLEMENTS/TABS 💊

EXERCISE/YOGA/ACTIVITY 🏃

_____   _____
_____   _____
_____   _____
_____   _____
_____   _____

SYMPTOMS/CRAVINGS/RESPONSE 🧍   ⚡ 🔋

_____
_____
_____

DATE: _____ CYCLE DAY : ☐ ⬙ MOOD: ☺ ☺ 😐 ☹ ☹

🌙 SLEPT FROM ___:___ TO ___:___   TOTAL HOURS : _____

I AM THANKFUL FOR ... 🙏
1._____
2._____
3._____

What did you eat today? 🍽

BREAKFAST	LUNCH	DINNER

SNACKS

Nutrition check list:

4 Proteins ☐   2 Fruits ☐   Nuts ☐
3 Veggies ☐   2 Carb ☐   Seeds ☐

Water: ⬛⬛⬛⬛⬛⬛⬛⬛⬛⬛⬛

🧘 : ☐   ⚖ _____

SUPPLEMENTS/TABS 💊   EXERCISE/YOGA/ACTIVITY 🏃

_____   _____
_____   _____
_____   _____
_____   _____
_____   _____

SYMPTOMS/CRAVINGS/RESPONSE 🧍   ⚡ 🔋

_____
_____
_____

DATE: _____ CYCLE DAY : ☐ ◇ MOOD: 😀 🙂 😐 🙁 😣

🌙💤 SLEPT FROM ___:___ TO ___:___ TOTAL HOURS : _____

I AM THANKFUL FOR ... 🙏

1. _____

2. _____

3. _____

What did you eat today? 🍽

BREAKFAST	LUNCH	DINNER

SNACKS

Nutrition check list:

4 Proteins ☐   2 Fruits ☐   Nuts ☐

3 Veggies ☐   2 Carb ☐   Seeds ☐

Water: 🥛🥛🥛🥛🥛🥛🥛🥛🥛🥛🥛

🧘 : ☐   ⚖

SUPPLEMENTS/TABS 💊   EXERCISE/YOGA/ACTIVITY 🏃

_____   _____
_____   _____
_____   _____
_____   _____
_____   _____

SYMPTOMS/CRAVINGS/RESPONSE 🔍   ⚡ 🔋

_____
_____
_____

DATE: _____ CYCLE DAY : ☐ ⬦ MOOD: 😀 🙂 😐 🙁 😣

🌙 SLEPT FROM ___:___ TO ___:___ TOTAL HOURS : _____

I AM THANKFUL FOR ... 🙏
1. _____
2. _____
3. _____

What did you eat today? 🍽

BREAKFAST	LUNCH	DINNER

SNACKS

Nutrition check list:

| 4 Proteins | ☐ | 2 Fruits | ☐ | Nuts | ☐ |
| 3 Veggies | ☐ | 2 Carb | ☐ | Seeds | ☐ |

Water: 🥛🥛🥛🥛🥛🥛🥛🥛🥛🥛

🧘 : ☐   ⚖

SUPPLEMENTS/TABS 💊   EXERCISE/YOGA/ACTIVITY 🏃

_____   _____
_____   _____
_____   _____
_____   _____
_____   _____

SYMPTOMS/CRAVINGS/RESPONSE 🧍   ⚡ 🔋

_____
_____
_____

Notes & Assessment

Notes & Assessment

Notes & Assessment

Printed in Great Britain
by Amazon

56344233R00061